Diabetes mellitus

(Types - Mechanisms – Complications)

Ayman Mohamed

ISBN: 1522985093
ISBN-13: 978-1522985099

DEDICATION

I dedicate my book to my family and many friends. A special feeling of gratitude to my loving parents, Saber Mohamed and Karema Ramadan, whose words of encouragement and push for tenacity ring in my ears. I dedicate this work and give special thanks to my aunt Dr. Sohair R. Fahmi

CONTENTS

ACKNOWLEDGMENTS

Firstly, I thank Allah for his grace, his success and his generosity.
I take this opportunity to express my profound gratitude and deep regards to Dr. Sohair R. Fahmi, Associate Professor of Physiology, Zoology Department, Faculty of Science, Cairo University, for supervising the present work, his guidance, monitoring and constant encouragement during the work.
I would like to express my sincere gratitude to Dr. Amel Mahmoud Ali Soliman, Associate Professor of Physiology, Zoology Department, Faculty of Science, Cairo University, for her supervision, valuable advices, stimulating suggestions through this work.
Special thanks to Prof. Dr. Mohamed Assem Said Marie, Professor of Environmental Physiology, Zoology Department, Faculty of Science, Cairo University, for his help and support.
I deeply thank my family for their love, support and encouragement through the work.

CHAPTER 1: GLUCOSE HOMEOSTASIS

Glucose is an essential metabolic substrate of all mammalian cells. Most of the energy needed to sustain life is delivered by oxidation of glucose . Glucose homeostasis represents the outcome of a complex feedback system for maintaining glucose tolerance within rather narrow physiological limits. In healthy individuals, glucose homeostasis is maintained by an insulin-regulated balance between glucose input to and removal from the blood stream. Defects in insulin secretion, insulin action or both pathways lead to development of chronic hyperglycaemia and finally overt diabetes.

The pancreas is considered as a doubled-entity organ, with both an exocrine and an endocrine component, reciprocally interacting in a composed system whose function is relevant for digestion, absorption, and homeostasis of nutrients. Pancreatic islets composed of many types of cells, including insulin-producing β cells, glucagon-releasing α cells, somatostatin-producing δ cells, pancreatic polypeptide-containing PP cells and ghrelin containing ε cells. All of these hormones are involved in the regulation of nutrient metabolism and glucose homeostasis. The defects in insulin secretion, insulin action, or both lead to loss of glucose homeostasis, with disturbances of carbohydrate, fat, and protein metabolism, which are the main features of the diabetes mellitus (DM) disease.

Normal Glucose Homeostasis

Glucose, a fundamental source of cellular energy, is released by the breakdown of endogenous glycogen stores that are primarily located in the liver. Glucose is also released indirectly in the muscle through intermediary metabolites. These whole-body energy stores are replenished from dietary glucose, which, after being digested and absorbed across the gut wall, is distributed among the various tissues of the body. Although glucose is required by all cells, its main consumer is the brain in the fasting or postabsorptive phase, which accounts for approximately 50% of the body's glucose use. Another 25% of glucose disposal occurs in the splanchnic area (liver and gastrointestinal tissue), and the remaining 25% takes place in insulin-dependent tissues, including muscles and adipose tissues . Approximately 85% of endogenous glucose production is derived from the liver, with glycogenolysis (conversion of glycogen to glucose) and gluconeogenesis (glucose formation) contributing equally to the basal rate of hepatic glucose production. The remaining ~15% of glucose is produced by the kidneys.

Normally, following glucose ingestion, the increase in plasma glucose concentration triggers insulin release, which stimulates splanchnic and peripheral glucose uptake and suppresses endogenous (primarily hepatic) glucose production. In healthy adults, blood glucose levels are tightly regulated within a range of 70 to 99 mg/dL, and maintained by specific hormones (eg, insulin, glucagon, incretins) as well as the central and peripheral nervous system, to meet metabolic requirements. Various cells and tissues (within the brain, muscles, gastrointestinal tract, liver, kidney, and adipose tissue) are also involved in blood glucose regulation by means of uptake, metabolism, storage, and excretion (Fig. 1).

This highly controlled process of glucose regulation may be particularly evident during the postprandial period, during which, under normal physiologic circumstances, glucose levels rarely rise beyond 140 mg/dL, even after consumption of a high-carbohydrate meal. Among the various hormones involved in glucose regulation, insulin and glucagon are the most relevant. Insulin, a potent antilipolytic (inhibiting fat breakdown) hormone, is known to reduce blood glucose levels by accelerating transport of glucose into insulin-sensitive cells and facilitating its conversion to storage compounds via glycogenesis (conversion of glucose to glycogen) and lipogenesis (fat formation). Glucagon, which also plays a central role in glucose homeostasis, is produced in response to low normal glucose levels or hypoglycemia and acts to increase glucose levels by accelerating glycogenolysis and promoting gluconeogenesis. After a glucose-containing meal, however, glucagon secretion is inhibited by hyperinsulinemia, which contributes to suppression of hepatic glucose production and maintenance of normal postprandial glucose tolerance.

The hormone amylin contributes to reduction in postprandial glucagon, as well as modest slowing of gastric emptying. Incretins, which include glucose-dependent insulinotropic polypeptide (GIP) and glucagon-like peptide-1 (GLP-1), are also involved in regulation of blood glucose, in part by their effects on insulin and glucagon. However, both GLP-1 and GIP are considered glucose-dependent hormones, meaning that they are secreted only when glucose levels raise above normal fasting plasma glucose levels; they do not directly stimulate insulin secretion. Normally, these hormones are released in response to meals and, by activating certain receptors (G protein–coupled) on pancreatic β-cells, they aid in stimulation of insulin secretion. When glucose levels are low, however, GLP1 and GIP levels (and their stimulating effects on insulin secretion) are diminished.

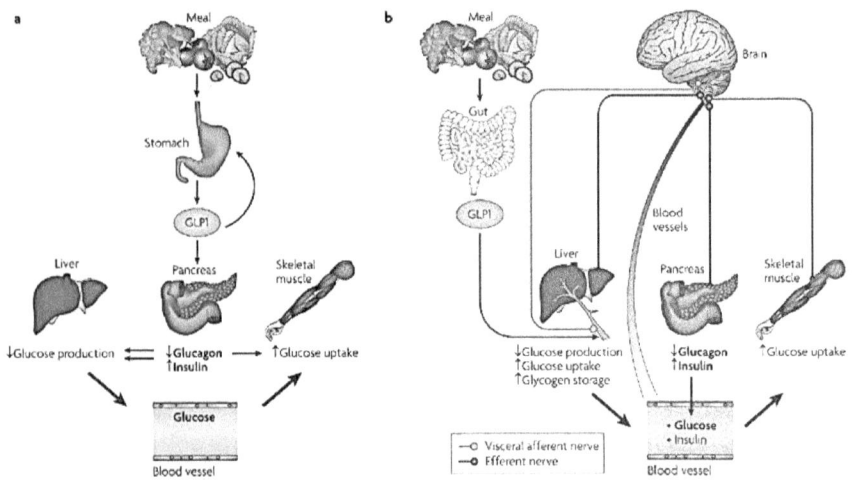

Nature Reviews | Drug Discovery

Fig. 1: (a) The endocrine regulation of glucose homeostasis at the three major peripheral sites: the liver, the pancreas and skeletal muscle. (b) The neuronal input to the central nervous system (CNS). In response to a

Cellular Uptake of Glucose

Since glucose cannot readily diffuse through cell membranes, it requires assistance from both insulin and a family of transport proteins (facilitated glucose transporter (GLUT) molecules) in order to gain entry into most cells. Essentially, GLUTs act as shuttles, forming an aqueous pore across hydrophobic cellular membranes, through which glucose can move more easily. The GLUT4 is a major mediator of glucose removal from the circulation and a key regulator of whole-body glucose homeostasis. Activation of GLUT4 and, in turn, facilitated glucose diffusion into muscle and adipose tissues, is dependent on the presence of insulin, whereas the function of other GLUTs is more independent on insulin. Once glucose enters the cells, it is phosphorylated (via glucokinase in the liver and hexokinase in most other cells), after which it cannot diffuse out of the cells and can then be either used for energy production or converted to a storage compounds (Fig. 2).

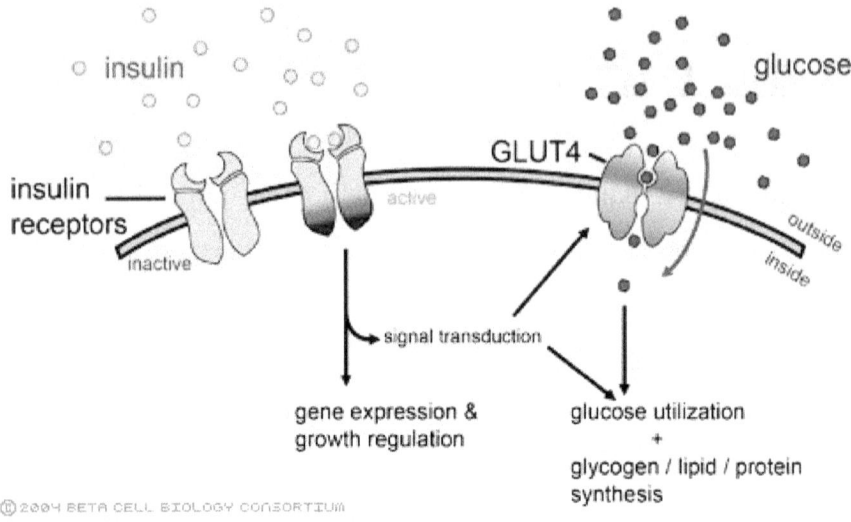

Fig. 2: Glucose transport into the cell.

Major Systems Involved in Glucose Utilization and Regulation

The majority of glucose uptake in peripheral tissues occurs in muscles, where glucose may either be used immediately for energy or stored as glycogen. As stated previously, transport of glucose into muscles is insulin-dependent, and thus requires insulin for activation of the major enzyme (glycogen synthase) that regulates production of glycogen. While adipose tissue is responsible for a much smaller amount of peripheral glucose uptake (2%-5%), it plays an important role in the maintenance of total body glucose homeostasis by regulating the release of free fatty acids (which increase gluconeogenesis) from stored triglycerides, influencing insulin sensitivity in the muscles and liver. While the liver does not require insulin to facilitate glucose uptake, it needs insulin to regulate glucose output. So, for example, when insulin concentrations are low, hepatic glucose output rises. Additionally, insulin helps the liver to store most of the absorbed glucose in the form of glycogen (Fig. 3).

The kidneys are increasingly recognized to play an important role in glucose homeostasis via release of glucose into the circulation (gluconeogenesis), uptake of glucose from the circulation to meet renal energy needs, and reabsorption of glucose at the proximal tubule. The kidneys also aid in elimination of excess glucose (when levels exceed approximately 180 mg/dL, though this threshold may rise during chronic hyperglycemia) by facilitating its excretion in the urine.

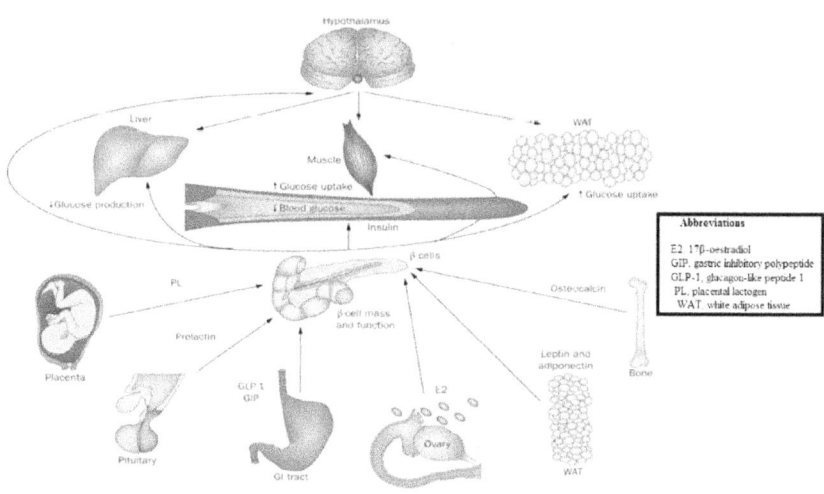

Fig. 3: Effect of hormones on glucose homeostasis.

Pancreatic β cells are critical to glucose homeostasis in the fed state, as they release insulin into the circulation, which stimulates glucose metabolism in liver, muscle, and white adipose tissue and brain cells. Other organs also modulate β cell mass and function via secreted hormones that act on β cell receptors to adapt them to physiological changes or metabolic stresses.

Impaired Glucose Tolerance/Impaired Fasting Glucose (IGT/IFG)

Pre-diabetes is an asymptomatic condition preceding diabetes including both impaired glucose tolerance (IGT) and impaired fasting glucose (IFG) and refers to blood glucose levels higher than normal but not reaching the level at which diabetes is diagnosed. IFG is defined as fasting plasma glucose (FPG) values of 100–125 mg/dl. (Normal fasting glucose level <100 mg/dl.) IGT is defined as 2 hr postprandial plasma glucose (PPG) of 140–199 mg/dl. (Normal 2 hr postprandial glucose level <140 mg/dl). Peoples with IGT or IFG are at significant risk for diabetes.

CHAPTER 2: DIABETES MELLITUS

Diabetes mellitus (DM) is a metabolic disorder resulting from a defect in insulin secretion, insulin action, or both. Insulin deficiency in turn leads to chronic hyperglycaemia with disturbances of carbohydrate, fat and protein metabolism. As the disease progresses tissue or vascular damage ensues leading to severe diabetic complications such as retinopathy, neuropathy, nephropathy, cardiovascular complications and ulceration. Thus, uncontrolled diabetes is implicated in a wide range of heterogeneous diseases.

Risk Factors

The risk factors for diabetes include family history of diabetes, body mass index (BMI) greater than 25 kg per m2, sedentary lifestyle, hypertension, dyslipidemia, history of gestational diabetes or large-for-gestational-age infant, and polycystic ovary syndrome.

Prevalence and Economic Effects

Diabetes mellitus (DM) is considered as one of the most dreaded metabolic disorders in the world. It is a complex and potentially debilitating disease that affects an estimated 8.3% of the adult population or 382 million people worldwide (Fig. 4). The region with the highest number of adults with diabetes (138 million) is the Western Pacific, which includes the People's Republic of China. It is estimated that 29.1 million people in the USA (9.3% of the population) have diabetes. If current trends continue, it is estimated that 592 million people worldwide will have diabetes by 2035.

Diabetes care has a major economic impact in both developed and developing countries. Estimated global health care costs to treat and prevent diabetes were at least $548 billion in 2011. In the USA, the total cost of diabetes was estimated to be $245 billion in 20122 and may exceed $500 billion by 2025.

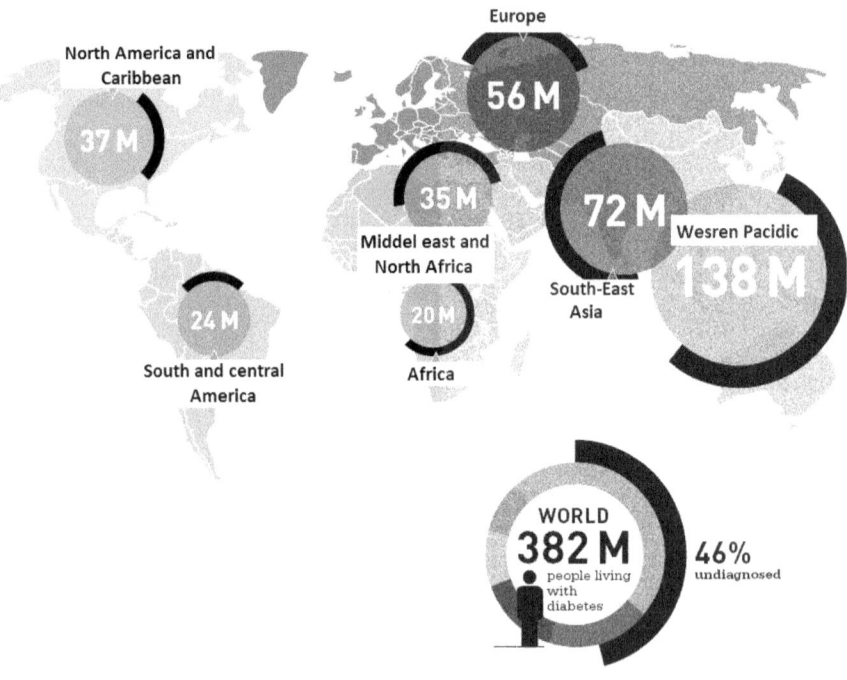

Fig. 4: Prevalence of diabetes.

Types of Diabetes Mellitus

1. Type 1 Diabetes Mellitus

Type 1diabetes (T1DM) is an autoimmune disease, which characterized by loss of insulin producing β cells and reliance on exogenous insulin for survival. The genetic factors alone does not lead to T1D, but the environmental factors also play a pivotal role as, viral infection, nitrosamine compounds, pre-eclampsia, and lack of vitamin A and/or D. T1DM is characterized by mononuclear infiltration of the pancreatic islets, followed by the destruction of insulin-producing β cells .

The two main forms of clinical type 1 diabetes are type 1a (about 90% of type 1 cases in Europe) which is thought to be due to immunological destruction of pancreatic β cells resulting in insulin deficiency; and type 1b (idiopathic, about 10% of type 1 diabetes), in which there is no evidence of autoimmunity. Type 1a is characterized by the presence of islet cell antibody (ICA), anti-glutamic acid decarboxylate (anti-GAD insulinoma-associated protein-2 (IA-2) that identify the autoimmune process with β cells destruction. Autoimmune diseases such as Grave's disease, Hashimoto's thyroiditis and Addison's disease may be associated with type 1 diabetes mellitus.

There is no known etiological basis for type 1b diabetes mellitus. Some of these patients have permanent insulinopaenia and are prone to ketoacidosis, but have no evidence of

11

autoimmunity. This form is more prevalent among individuals of African and Asian Origin.

2. <u>Type 2 Diabetes Mellitus</u>

Type 2 diabetes mellitus (T2DM) accounts for 90, 95% diabetic patients. T2DM is increasing in prevalence worldwide, and it is strongly associated with obesity and insulin resistance, as well as defects in pancreatic β cells function and mass. It is a multifactorial disease, where the pathophysiology of which involves not only the pancreas, but also the liver, skeletal muscle, adipose tissue, gastrointestinal tract, brain, and kidney.

Current theories of type 2 diabetes include a defect in insulin-mediated glucose uptake in muscle, a dysfunction of the pancreatic β-cells, a disruption of secretory function of adipocytes, and an impaired insulin action in liver. Reduced sensitivity to insulin in liver, muscle, and adipose tissue, and a progressive decline in pancreatic β-cell function leading to impaired insulin secretion, eventually result in hyperglycemia, the hallmark feature of T2DM . The etiology of human type 2 diabetes is multifactorial with genetic background and environmental factors of the modern world which favor the development of obesity. Several findings indicate that genetics is an important contributing factor. It has been estimated that 30 – 70% of type 2 diabetes risk can be attributed to genetics. The lifetime risk of T2DM is about 7% in a general population, about 40% in offspring of one parent with T2DM, and about 70% if both parents have T2DM. Patterns of inheritance suggest that T2DM is both polygenic and heterogeneous – i.e. multiple genes are involved and different combinations of genes play a role in different subsets of individuals. Genetic research effort have led to the identification of at least 27 T2DM susceptibility genes and most recent genome-wide association studies have identified 20 common genetic variants associated with T2DM.

Since skeletal muscles account for ~ 75% of whole body insulin-stimulated glucose uptake, defects in this tissue play a major role in glucose homeostasis in patients with T2DM.

Insulin resistance may be defined as a condition in which normal insulin concentrations fail to achieve a normal metabolic response. Insulin resistance is usually characterized by a reduction in insulin-stimulated storage of glucose as glycogen in skeletal muscle and liver. Insulin resistance in skeletal muscles is among the earliest detectable defects in humans with T2DM. Type 2 diabetic patients are characterized by a decreased fat oxidative capacity and high levels of circulating free fatty acid. The latter is known to cause insulin resistance by reducing stimulated glucose uptake most likely via accumulation of lipid inside the muscle cells. A reduced fat oxidative capacity and metabolic inflexibility are important components of skeletal muscles insulin resistance.

3. <u>Gestational Diabetes Mellitus</u>

Gestational diabetes mellitus is defined as "carbohydrate

intolerance with onset or first recognition during pregnancy" . This definition includes pregnancies in which the following occur: insulin therapy is required, diabetes persists after delivery, and diabetes may have been present, but not recognized, prior to the pregnancy. Women at risk of T2DM are at risk of gestational DM. Gestational DM is a heterogeneous disorder in which age, obesity, and genetic background contribute to the severity of the disease. Multiparous women have a very high prevalence of gestational diabetes mellitus. There has been relatively little research in the area of gestational diabetes genetics.There is evidence for clustering of T2DM and impaired glucose tolerance in families with gestational DM and evidence for higher prevalence of T2DM in mothers of women with gestational DM.

The pathophysiology of gestational diabetes remains controversial. Gestational DM may reflect a predisposition to T2DM under the metabolic conditions of pregnancy or it may represent the extreme manifestation of metabolic alterations that normally occur in pregnancy. Women with gestational diabetes have decreased insulin sensitivity in comparison with control groups. Gestational diabetes induces a state of dyslipidemia consistent with insulin resistance. During pregnancy, women with gestational diabetes have high serum triacylglycerol concentrations but lower LDL-cholesterol concentrations than healthy pregnant women . During pregnancy, gestational diabetes is associated with a number of complications for child. Because insulin does not cross the placenta, the fetus is exposed to the maternal hyperglycemia. The fetal pancreas is capable of responding to this hyperglycemia. The fetus becomes hyperinsulinemic, which in turn promotes growth and subsequent macrosomia (newborn with an excessive birth weight).

Fetus born to mother with gestational diabetes has higher risk of developing macrosomia, neonatal hypoglycemia, hyperbilirubinemia, shoulder dystonia with its attendant risk of brachial injury and clavicle fracture. These complications have been reported with varying frequency. Additionally, there are some data that suggest an increase in fetal malformation and perinatal mortality. Cesarean sections are also more common, and gestational DM is associated with a higher risk of pre-eclampsia. Infant exposed to maternal diabetes in uterus have an increased risk of diabetes and obesity in childhood and adulthood. Studies have indicated that the magnitude of fetal-neonatal risk of diabetes and obesity in childhood and adulthood is proportional to the severity of maternal hyperglycemia. Gestational DM is one of the most common complications in pregnancy occurring in 2, 20 % - 8, 80 % of each year, dependent on the ethnic mix of the population and the criteria used for diagnosis.

4. <u>Maturity Onset Diabetes of Young (MODY)</u>

MODY is a monogenic and autosomal dominant form of diabetes mellitus. The disease was described in 1974 – 1975 and since then newer gene mutations and subgroups of MODY have been identified. To distinguish MODY from type 1 diabetes tests needs to be done to establish the absence of diabetes antibodies (anti-insulin, anti-islet, anti-glutamic acid decarboxylase). In obese people, the absence of insulin resistance will differentiate it from T2DM.

MODY presents in children, adolescents or young adults and may account for up to 5% of diabetes cases. MODY patients have a strong family history of diabetes, suggestive of a primary genetic cause. MODY is caused by changes to a single gene and if either one of the parent carriers, this gene they have a 50% chance of passing it on to their child. Disease progression in MODY is thought to be largely independent of nongenetic factors other than time. Nine of genetic forms of MODY have been identified to date, and these have been termed MODY 1 – 9. These rare diabetic disorders are associated with heterozygosity for mutations in single genes, including 7 transcription factors (MODY 1, 3, 4, 5, 6, 7 and 9) and 2 metabolic enzymes (MODY 2 and 8).

5. <u>Neonatal Diabetes Mellitus</u>

Neonatal diabetes mellitus is defined as insulin-sensitive hyperglycemia occurring in the first months of life, lasting for more than 2 weeks and required insulin for management . It is rare, with an incidence of approximately 1 in 500 000 births. Neonatal diabetes mellitus is considered distinct from autoimmune type 1 diabetes, which manifests after the first 3 to 6 months of life. In this disease, antibodies to insulin or islet cells and other markers of autoimmune T1DM are absent. There are two separate forms of neonatal diabetes mellitus that vary in the length of insulin dependency in the premature stage of disease. In about 50% of cases of neonatal diabetes mellitus, diabetes is transient and resolves at a median age of 3 months (Transient Neonatal Diabetes Mellitus). The other 50% of cases of neonatal diabetes mellitus are permanent (Permanent Neonatal Diabetes Mellitus).

The etiology of neonatal diabetes mellitus is genetically heterogeneous, producing abnormal development or absence of pancreas or islets, decreased β-cell mass secondary to increased β cell apoptosis, and β-cell dysfunction that limits insulin secretion. Transient neonatal diabetes mellitus is a form of neonatal diabetes that appears in the first six weeks of life and usually ends by 18 months. It is characterized by intrauterine growth retardation, dehydration, small gestational age at birth, and failure to thrive. Permanent neonatal diabetes mellitus can occur alone or as a larger genetic syndrome. In permanent neonatal diabetes mellitus, diabetes develops within days to months after birth and persists throughout life. Intrauterine growth retardation, hyperglycemia, severe dehydration, osmotic polyuria, and failure to thrive are all associated with permanent neonatal diabetes mellitus.

Assigning a type of diabetes to an individual often depends on the circumstances present at the time of diagnosis, and many diabetic individuals do not easily fit into a single class. For example, a person with gestational diabetes mellitus (GDM) may continue to be hyperglycemic after delivery and may be determined to have, in fact, T2DM. Alternatively, a person who acquires diabetes because of large doses of exogenous steroids may become normoglycemic once the glucocorticoids are discontinued, but then may develop diabetes many years later after recurrent episodes of pancreatitis.

Symptoms of Diabetes Mellitus

Symptoms are similar in the different types of diabetes but they vary in their intensity (Fig. 5). Symptoms develop more rapidly in T1DM and more typical. The primary symptoms of diabetes include diuresis, thirst and tiredness. These are a result of the entrance of glucose to the urine when the renal threshold for glucose reabsorption is exceeded. An osmotic diuresis is developed resulting in dehydration and the following thirst. Diabetes is also associated with a disturbed fat metabolism. When insulin is absent, fat is broken down to acetyl-CoA via beta-oxidation. The excess acetyl-CoA is further converted into ketone bodies, which is leading to ketosis.

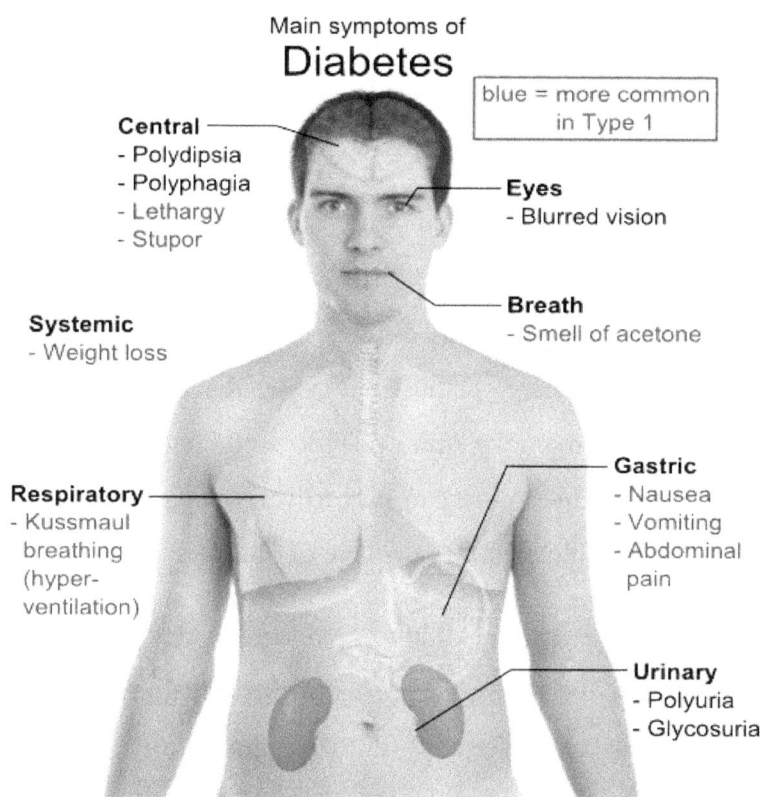

Main symptoms of
Diabetes

blue = more common
in Type 1

Central
- Polydipsia
- Polyphagia
- Lethargy
- Stupor

Eyes
- Blurred vision

Breath
- Smell of acetone

Systemic
- Weight loss

Gastric
- Nausea
- Vomiting
- Abdominal
  pain

Respiratory
- Kussmaul
  breathing
  (hyper-
  ventilation)

Urinary
- Polyuria
- Glycosuria

Fig. 5: Symptoms of diabetes mellitus

CHAPTER 3: DIABETIC COMPLICATIONS

<u>Diabetic complications</u>

Diabetes is associated with a number of complications. Acute metabolic complications associated with mortality include diabetic ketoacidosis from exceptionally high blood glucose concentrations (hyperglycemia) and coma as the result of low blood glucose (hypoglycemia). These complications are wide ranging and are due at least in part to chronic elevation of blood glucose levels, which leads to damage of blood vessels.

In diabetes, the resulting complications are grouped under "microvascular disease" (due to damage of small blood vessels) and "macrovascular disease" (due to damage of the arteries). Microvascular complications include eye disease or "retinopathy," kidney disease termed "nephropathy," and neural damage or "neuropathy". The major macrovascular complications include accelerated cardiovascular disease resulting in myocardial infarction and cerebrovascular disease manifesting as strokes. Although the underlying etiology remains controversial, there is also myocardial dysfunction associated with diabetes which appears at least in part to be independent of atherosclerosis. Other chronic complications of diabetes include depression, dementia, and sexual dysfunction.

1. <u>Nephropathy</u>

Diabetic nephropathy represents the major cause of end stage renal failure in Western societies. Clinically, it is characterized by the development of proteinuria with a subsequent decline in glomerular filtration rate, which progresses over a long period of time, often over 10–20 years. If left untreated, the resulting uremia is fatal .

Importantly, kidney disease is also a major risk factor for the development of macrovascular complications such as heart attacks and strokes. Hypertension and poor glycemic control frequently precede overt diabetic nephropathy, although a subset of patients develop nephropathy despite good glycemic control and normal blood pressure. Once nephropathy is established, blood pressure is often seen to rise, but paradoxically in the short term, there can be improvements in glycemic control as a result of reduced renal insulin clearance by the kidney.

2. <u>Retinopathy</u>

Diabetic retinopathy is characterized by a spectrum of lesions within the retina and is the leading cause of blindness among adults aged 20–74 years. These include changes in vascular permeability, capillary microaneurysms, capillary degeneration, and excessive formation of new blood vessels (neovascularization). The neural retina is also dysfunctional with death of some cells, which alters retinal electrophysiology and results in an inability to discriminate between colors.

Clinically, diabetic retinopathy is separated into nonproliferative and proliferative disease stages. In the early stages, hyperglycemia can lead to intramural pericyte death and thickening of the basement membrane, which contribute to changes in the integrity of blood vessels within the retina, altering the blood-retinal barrier and vascular permeability. In this initial stage of nonproliferative diabetic retinopathy (NPDR), most people do not notice any visual impairment.

Degeneration or occlusion of retinal capillaries are strongly associated with worsening prognosis, which is most likely the result of ischemia followed by subsequent release of angiogenic factors including those related to hypoxia. This progresses the disease into the proliferative phase where neovascularization and accumulation of fluid within the retina, termed macula edema, contribute to visual impairment. In more severe cases, there can be bleeding with associated distorting of the retinal architecture including development of a fibrovascular membrane which can subsequently lead to retinal detachment.

3. **Neuropathy**

Diabetic neuropathy affects all peripheral nerves, including pain fibers, motor neurons and the autonomic nervous system. The pathogenesis of diabetic neuropathy is complicated, and the mechanism of this disease remains poorly understood. It has been suggested that hyperglycemia is responsible for changes in the nerve tissue. Changes in the blood vessels supplying the peripheral nerves underlie the mechanisms involved in microvascular damage and hypoxia. These changes are based on increases in wall thickness with the hyalinization of the vessel walls and the basal lamina of arterioles and capillaries, leading to nerve ischemia. Through revised primary capillary membrane to the endoneurium penetrates the plasma protein, causing swelling and increased interstitial pressure in the nerves as well as capillary pressure, fibrin deposition and thrombus formation.

More than half of all individuals with diabetes eventually develop neuropathy, with a lifetime risk of one or more lower extremity amputations estimated in some populations to be up to 15%. Diabetic neuropathy is a syndrome which encompasses both the somatic and autonomic divisions of the peripheral nervous system. There is, however, a growing appreciation that damage to the spinal cord and the higher central nervous system can also occur. Disease progression in neuropathy was traditionally clinically characterized by the development of vascular abnormalities, such as capillary basement membrane thickening and endothelial hyperplasia with subsequent diminishment in oxygen tension and hypoxia. Inhibitors of the renin-angiotensin system and α-1 antagonists improve nerve conduction velocities in the clinical context, which is postulated to be a result of increases in neuronal blood flow.

Advanced neuropathy due to nerve fiber deterioration in diabetes is characterized by altered sensitivities to vibrations and thermal thresholds, which progress to loss of sensory perception. Hyperalgesia, paresthesias, and allodynia also occur in a proportion of patients, with pain evident in 40–50% of those with diabetic neuropathy. Pain is also seen in some diabetic individuals without clinical evidence of neuropathy (10–20%), which can seriously impede quality of life.

4. <u>Cardiovascular Diseases</u>

There is increased risk of cardiovascular disease (CVD) in diabetes, such that an individual with diabetes has a risk of myocardial infarction equivalent to that of nondiabetic individuals who have previously had a myocardial infarction. CVD accounts for more than half of the mortality seen in the diabetic population, and diabetes equates to an approximately threefold increased risk of myocardial infarction compared with the general population . In type 1 diabetes, it is not common to see progression to CVD without impairment in kidney function . In type 2 diabetes, kidney disease remains a major risk factor for premature CVD, in addition to dyslipidemia, poor glycemic control, and persistent elevations in blood pressure. Cardiovascular disorders in diabetes include premature atherosclerosis, manifest as myocardial infarction and stroke as well as impaired cardiac function, predominantly diastolic dysfunction.

CHAPTER 4: MECHANISMS OF DIABETIC COMPLICATIONS

1. <u>Oxidative Stress</u>

Oxidative stress is currently suggested as the mechanism underlying diabetes and diabetic complications. Metabolic disorders, assist the increased reactive oxygen species (ROS) production in the physiological system such as obesity, insulin resistance and diabetes mellitus. ROS overproduction above the physiological level can overcome the functions of the cellular antioxidant system, leading to oxidative stress. Hyperglycemia condition can induce oxidative stress by several mechanisms such as glucose autoxidation, polyol pathway, advanced glycation endproduct AGE) formation and protein kinase C (PKC). These free radicals are formed through non-enzymatic glycation reactions, mitochondrial electron transport chain dysfunctions or activation of hexoseamines in the presence of hyperglycemia (Fig. 6).

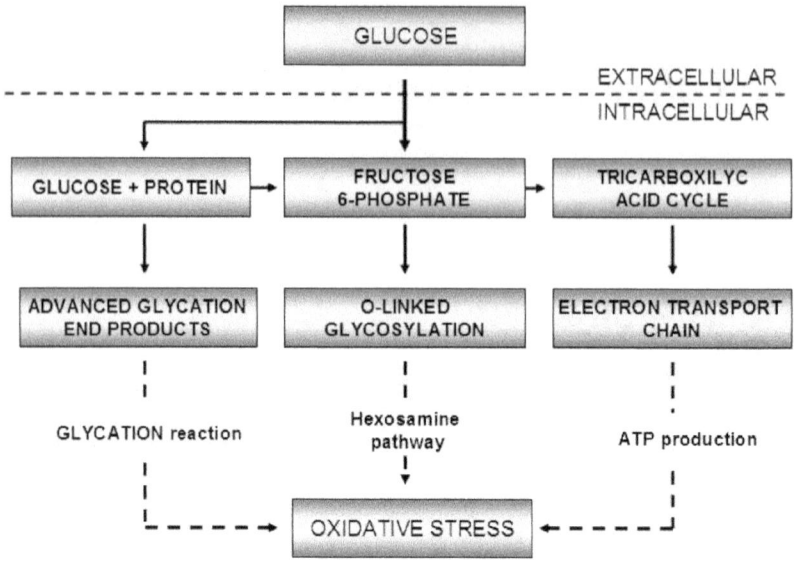

Fig. 6: The link between oxidative stress and diabetes.

ROS disrupt transmission pathways between the insulin receptor and the glucose transport system, which leads to an onset in insulin resistance and are involved also in the inactivation of the two critical anti-atherosclerotic enzymes: endothelial nitric oxide and prostacyclin synthase. ROS not only participate in the formation of advanced glycated end products (AGE), but also mediate AGE effects on target tissues. The connection between clinical complications of DM and oxidative stress arises from the formation of high doses of AGE in this metabolic disorder.

2. <u>Advanced Glycated End Products</u>

Advanced glycation end products (AGEs) are modifications of proteins or lipids that become nonenzymatically glycated and oxidized after contact with aldose sugars. Early glycation and oxidation processes result in the formation of Schiff bases and Amadori products. Further glycation of proteins and lipids causes molecular rearrangements that lead to the generation of AGEs (Fig. 7).

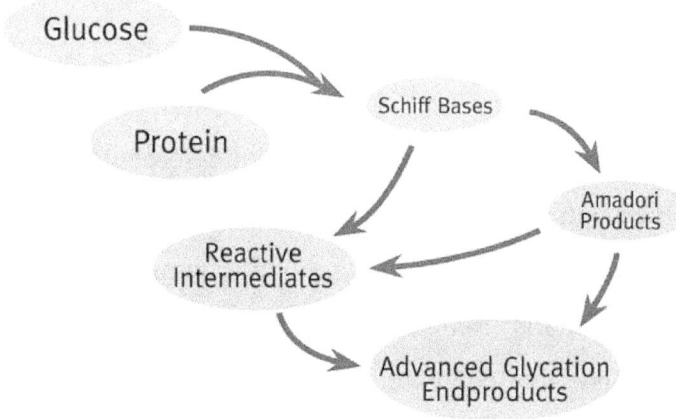

Fig. 7: Formation of AGEs.

AGEs may fluoresce, produce reactive oxygen species (ROS), bind to specific cell surface receptors, and form cross-links. AGEs form *in vivo* in hyperglycemic environments and during aging and contribute to the pathophysiology of vascular disease in diabetes.

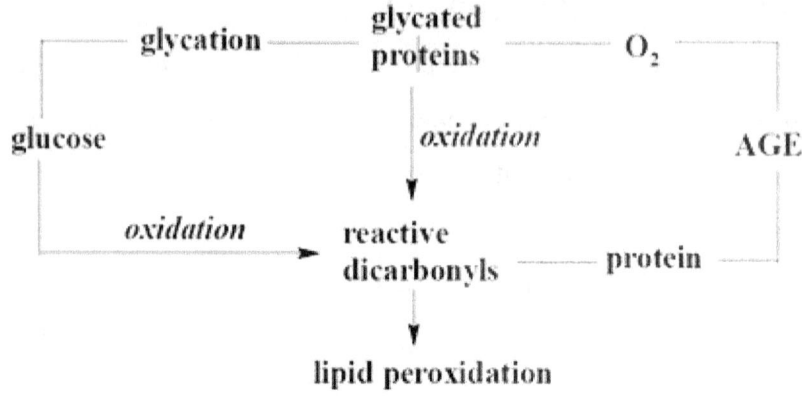

Fig. 8: The relation between ROS and AGEs.

AGEs induce link processes in the structure of long lifespan proteins, such as collagen, modifying blood vessel structure. By binding to their specific receptors (RAGEs), they activate intracellular signaling pathways which lead to cytokine production, responsible for the proinflammatory and prosclerotic effects. TAGEs (toxic AGEs), derived from glyceraldehydes, are very aggressive compounds and represent the dominant form of AGEs. The interaction between TAGEs and their receptors in endothelial and inflammatory cells, leads to intracellular generation of reactive oxygen species (ROS) via the electron transport chain, NADPH oxidase, xanthine oxidase and arachidonic acid metabolism (Fig. 8).

3. Aldose Reductase Pathway

Aldose reductase (AR) participates in the glucose

28

metabolism by being the rate-limiting enzyme of the polyol (polyhydric alcohol) pathway. In this pathway glucose is reduced to sorbitol by AR, using NADPH as an electron donor. Sorbitol is subsequently oxidized to fructose by the enzyme sorbitol dehydrogenase (SDH), using nicotinamide adenine dinucleotide (NAD+) as an electron acceptor (Fig. 9).

The polyol pathway

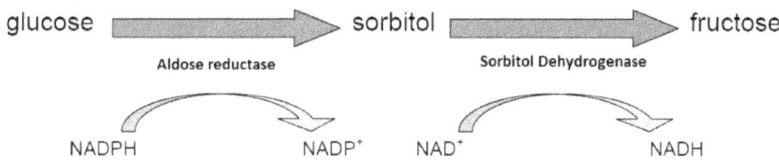

Fig. 9: The polyol pathway

During euglycemic conditions the main task of the polyol pathway is to provide sorbitol to balance the osmotic pressure in the renal medulla and to produce fructose as an energy source for sperm in the seminal vesicle.

AR acts on many different aldehyde-containing substrates but sugars with shorter chains are better substrates than hexoses. Due to its low affinity for glucose, only 3% of all glucose is converted to sorbitol at normal glucose levels. Instead, glucose is mainly phosphorylated into glucose 6-phosphate by hexokinase, which is further metabolized to pyruvate and lactate via the glycolytic pathway. During hyperglycemias conditions, however, one third of the glucose is metabolized by the polyol pathway. In addition, the AR activity is enhanced by high glucose concentrations. This hyperglycemia-induced increase in flux through the polyol pathway has been proposed to play an important role in the pathogenesis of secondary diabetic complications in the eyes, nerves and kidneys.

Although it is unknown how the increased flux through the polyol pathway is involved in the occurrence of diabetic disorders several possible mechanisms have been suggested. One of the first mechanisms proposed is based on the development of osmotic stress due to sorbitol accumulation. Glucose can easily penetrate the cell membrane while the polyol sorbitol is an osmolyte with low permeability. Thus, the excessive polyol pathway metabolism results in an accumulation of sorbitol inside the cells. This causes hypertonicity and osmotic imbalance that in turn leads to typical diabetic complications, due to swelling and disruption of the intracellular environment.

The most discussed explanation today to the deleterious effects of diabetes caused by a hyperactive polyol pathway is an increased oxidative stress. When the flux through the polyol pathway is enhanced the cofactor NADPH is depleted resulting in decreased regeneration of reduced glutathione (GSH), which also requires NADPH to be formed. GSH is a key player in this antioxidative system, with a significant function in ROS scavenging . The depletion of NADPH also affects the production of NO since NO synthase competes with AR for the same cofactor (Fig.10).

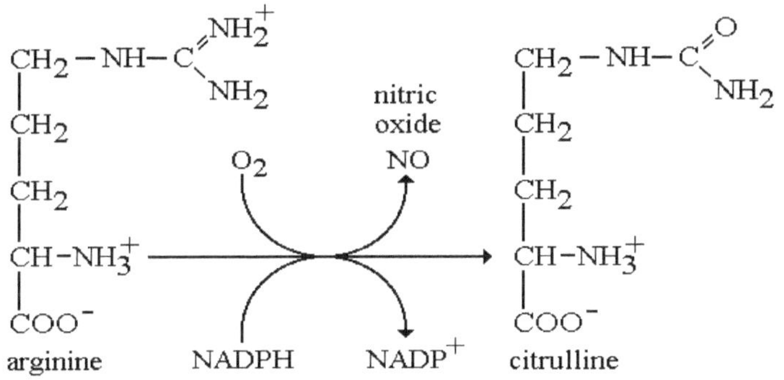

Fig. 10: Synthesis of NO.

Decreased levels of NO produce vasoconstriction and slowing of nerve conduction, which is involved in the pathogenesis of diabetic neuropathy. It has also been suggested that NOS is inactivated by enhanced levels of ROS, i.e. superoxide, produced as a result of the hyperglycemia increased endothelial cell sorbitol concentrations.

4. Protein Kinase Theory

Protein kinase C (PKC) comprises a family of at least 12 isoforms of serine threonine kinases. Many *in vivo* and *in vitro* studies have suggested that increased diacylglycerol (DAG) levels in vascular tissues, is related with PKC activation in diabetes mellitus (Fig. 11).

The source of DAG that activates PKC can be derived from

the hydrolysis of phosphatidylinositides (PIs) or from the metabolism ofphosphatidylcholine (PC) by phospholipase C (PLC) or phospholipase D (PLD). Alternatively, DAG can be synthesized by *de novo* pathway from glycolytic intermediates. In metabolic labeling studies, it has been reported that the incorporation of glucose into the glycerol backbone of DAG was increased by hyperglycemia, suggesting that increased DAG contents were partly derived from *de novo* pathway. Recent studies have identified that the activation of protein kinase C (PKC) and increased diacylglycerol (DAG) levels are associated with many vascular abnormalities in retinal, renal, and cardiovascular tissues.

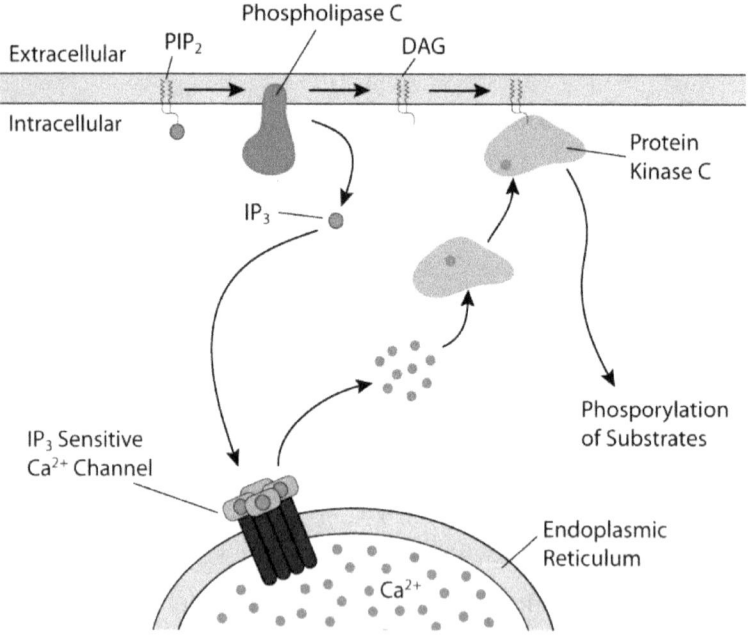

Fig.11: Activation of PKC.

REFERENCES

Abbott, C.A.; Malik, R.A.; van Ross, E.R.; Kulkarni, J. and Boulton, A.J. (2011): Prevalence and characteristics of painful diabetic neuropathy in a large community-based diabetic population in the UK. Diab. Care, 34: 2220–2224.

ADA. (2008): Economic costs of diabetes in the U.S. in 2007. Diab. Care, 31(3):596-615.

Adeniyi, A.F.; Adeleye, J.O. and Adeniyi, C.Y. (2011): Diabetes, sexual dysfunction and therapeutic exercise: a 20 year review. Curr. Diabetes Rev., 6: 201–206.

Aguilar-Bryan, L., and Bryan, J. (2008): Neonatal diabetes mellitus. Endocrine Reviews, 29(3): 265-291.

Ahrén, B. and Corrigan, C.B. (1984): Intermittent need for insulin in a subgroup of diabetic patients in Tanzania. Diabet. Med., 2: 262-264.

Amico, J.A. and Klein, I. (1981): Diabetic management in patients with renal failure. Diab. Care, 4: 430–434.

Ashafaq, M.; Varshney , L.; Khan, M.H.; Salman, M.; Naseem, M.; Wajid, S. and Parvez , S. (2014): Neuromodulatory effects of hesperidin in mitigating oxidative stress in streptozotocin induced diabetes. Biomed. Res. Int., 2014: 249031.

Assmann, A.; Hinault, C. and Kulkarni, R.N. (2009): Growth factor control of pancreatic islet regeneration and function. Pediatric. Diab., 10(1): 14–32.

Atkinson, M.A. and Maclaren, N.K. (1994): The pathogenesis of insulin-dependent diabetes mellitus. N. Engl. J. Med., 331: 1428-1436.

Avery, M.D. and Rossi M.A. (1994): Gestational diabetes. J. Nurse-Midwifery, 39(2): 9-19.

Bastaki, S. (2005): Diabetes mellitus and its treatment. Int. J. Diabetes Metabolism, 13:111-134

Bearse, M.A. Jr.; Han, T.; Schneck, M. E.; Barez, S.; Jacobsen, C. and Adams, A.J. (2004): Local multifocal oscillatory potential abnormalities in diabetes and early diabetic retinopathy. Invest. Ophthal. Vis. Sci., 45: 3259-3265.

Bhattacharya, S.; Manna, P.; Gachhui, R. and Sil, P.C. (2013): D-saccharic acid 1,4-lactone protects diabetic rat kidney by ameliorating hyperglycemia-mediated oxidative stress and renal inflammatory cytokines via NF-κB and PKC signaling. Toxicol. Appl. Pharmacol., 267:16–29.

Bjornholm , M. and Zierath J. (2005): Insulin signal transduction in human skeletal muscle: identifying the defects in type 2 diabetes. Biochem. Soc. Trans., 33(2): 354-357.

Black, E. E.; Wagenmakers, A. J.; Glatz, J.F.; Wolffenbuttel, B.H.; Kemerink, G.J.; Langenberg, C.J.; Heidendal, G.A. and Saris, W.H. (2000): Plasma FFA utilization and fatty acid binding protein content are diminished in type 2 diabetic muscle. Am. J. Physiol. Endocrinol. Metabol., 279(1):, 146-154.

Boden, G. (1999): Free fatty acids, insulin resistance, and type 2 diabetes mellitus. Proceed. Assoc. Am. Phys., 111(3): 241-248.

Bresnick, G.H.; Engerman, R.; Davis, M.D.; de Venecia, G. and Myers, F.L. (1976): Patterns of ischemia in diabetic retinopathy. Trans. Sect .Ophthalmol. Am. Acad. Ophthalmol. Otolaryngol., 81: 694–709.

Brownlee, M. (2005): The pathobiology of diabetic complications. A unifying mechanism. Diabetes, 54: 1615-1624.

Brownlee, M.; Vlassara, H. and Cerami, A. (1985): Nonenzymatic glycosylation products on collagen covalently trap low-density lipoprotein. Diabetes., 34: 938–941.

Bryant, N.J.; Govers, R. and James, D.E. (2002): Regulated transport of the glucose transporter GLUT4. Nat. Rev. Mol. Cell Biol., 3(4):267-277.

Butler, A. E.; Janson, J.; Bonner-Weir, S.; Ritzel, R.; Rizza, R. A. and Butler, P. C.(2003): Beta-cell deficit and increased beta-cell apoptosis in humans with type 2 diabetes. Diabetes, 52: 102–110.

Butte, N.F. (2000): Carbohydrate and lipid metabolism in pregnancy: normal compared with gestational diabetes mellitus. Am. J. Clin. Nutr., 71(5): 1256-1261.

Campbell, P.J.; Mandarino, L.J. andGerich, J.E. (1988): Quantification of the relative impairment in actions of insulin on hepatic glucose production and peripheral glucose uptake in non-insulin-dependent diabetes mellitus. Metabolism, 37:15-21.

Capes, S. and Anand, S. (2001): What is type 2 diabetes? In: Gerstein HC, Haynes RB, eds. Evidence-based diabetes care. Hamilton, Ont. Decker.,14:151–163.

CDCP. (2014): National diabetes statistics report: estimates of diabetes and its burden in the United States, 2014. Available from:

http://www.cdc.gov/diabetes/pubs/statsreport14/national-diabetes-report-web.pdf.

Cheung, N.W. (2009): The management of gestational diabetes. Vasc. Health Risk Manag., 5: 153-164.

Cornell, S. (2015): Continual evolution of type 2 diabetes: an update on pathophysiology and emerging treatment options. Ther Clin. Risk Manag., 16(11):621-632.

Cukierman, T.; Gerstein, H.C. and Williamson, J.D. (2005): Cognitive decline and dementia in diabetes– systematic overview of prospective observational studies. Diabetologia., 48: 2460–2469.

Czyzyk, A. (1987): Pathophysiology and diabetes clinic (Polish).

P.Z.W.L. Warszawa, 1987:146–147.

Damasceno, D.C.; Netto, A.O.; Iessi, I.L.; Gallego, F.Q.; Corvino, S.B.; Dallaqua, B.; Sinzato, Y.K.; Bueno, A.; Calderon, I.M. and Rudge, M.V. (2014): Streptozotocin-induced diabetes models: pathophysiological mechanisms and fetal . Biomed. Res. Int., 2014: 819065.

DCCTR. (1993): The effect of intensive treatment on the development and progression of long-term complications in insulindependent diabetes mellitus. N. Engl. J. Med., 329: 977–986.

DeFronzo, R.A. (2004): Diabetes: pathogenesis of type 2 diabetes mellitus. Med. Clin. N. Am.,88:787-835.

Domanski, M.; Mitchell, G.; Pfeffer, M.; Neaton, J.D.; Norman, J.; Svendsen, K.; Grimm, R.; Cohen, J. and Stamler, J. (2002): Pulse pressure and cardiovascular disease-related mortality: follow- up study of the Multiple Risk Factor Intervention Trial (MRFIT). JAMA., 287: 2677–2683.

Doria, A.; Patti, M-E. and Kahn, C.R. (2008): The emerging genetic architecture of type 2 diabetes. Cell Metab 8(3): 186-200.

Drucker, D.J. (2006): The biology of incretin hormones. Cell Metab.,3:153-165.

Drucker, D.J. and Nauck, M. (2006): The incretin system: glucagon-like peptide-1 receptor agonists and dipeptidyl peptidase-4 inhibitors in type 2 diabetes. Lancet, 368:1696-1705.

Drury, P.L.; Ting, R.; Zannino, D.; Ehnholm, C.; Flack, J.; Whiting, M.; Fassett, R.; Ansquer, J.C.; Dixon, P.; Davis, T.M.; Pardy, C.; Colman, P. and Keech, A. (2011): Estimated glomerular filtration rate and albuminuria are independent predictors of cardiovascular events and death in type 2 diabetes mellitus: the Fenofibrate Intervention and Event Lowering in Diabetes (FIELD) study. Diabetologia. 54: 32–43.

Ebaid, H. (2014): Promotion of immune and glycaemic functions in streptozotocin-induced diabetic rats treated with un-denatured camel milk whey proteins. Nutr. Metabol., 11:1-31.

Folli, F.; Corradi, D.; Fanti, P.; Davalli, A.; Paez, A.; Giaccari, A.; Perego, C. Diabetologia Muscogiuri, G. (2011): The Role of Oxidative Stress in the Pathogenesis of Type 2 Diabetes Mellitus Micro and Macrovascular Complications: Avenues for a Mechanistic-Based Therapeutic Approach. Current Diabetes Reviews., 7(5):313-324.

Forbes, J. M. and Cooper, M. E. (2011): Mechanisms of Diabetic Complications. Physiol. Rev., 93 (1): 137-188.

Frank, R.N. (2004): Diabetic retinopathy. N. Engl. J. Med., 350: 48–58.

Garner, P. (1995): Type 1 diabetes mellitus and pregnancy. Lancet, 346(8968): 157-161.

Genuthm, S.; Albertim, K.G.; Bennettm, P.; Busem, J.; Defronzo, R.; Kahn, R.; Kitzmiller, J.; Knowler, W.C.; Lebovitz, H.; Lernmark, A.; Nathan, D.; Palmer, J.; Rizza, R.; Saudek, C.; Shaw, J.; Steffes, M.; Stern, M.; Tuomilehto, J. and Zimmet, P. (2003): Expert Committee on the Diagnosis and Classification of Diabetes Mellitus. Follow-up report on the diagnosis of diabetes mellitus. Diab. Care, 26:3160–3167.

Gilbertson, D.T.; Liu, J.; Xue, J.L.; Louis, T.A.; Solid, C.A.; Ebben, J.P. and Collins, A.J. (2005): Projecting the number of patients with end-stage renal disease in the United States to the year 2015. J. Am. Soc. Nephrol., 16: 3736–3741.

Groop, P.H.; Thomas, M.C.; Moran, J.L.; Waden, J.; Thorn, L.M.; Makinen, V.P.; Rosengard-Barlund, M.; Saraheimo, M.; Hietala, K.; Heikkila, O. and Forsblom, C. (2009): The presence and severity of chronic kidney disease predicts all-cause mortality in type 1 diabetes. Diabetes 58: 1651–1658.

Guilherme, A.; Virbasius, J.V.; Puri, V. and Czech, M. P. (2008): Adipocyte dysfunctions linking obesity to insulin resistance and type 2 diabetes. Nat. Rev. Mol. Cell. Biol., 9(5):367-377.

Gupta, S.; Chough, E.; Daley, J.; Oates, P.; Tornheim, K.; Ruderman, N.B.; Keaney, J.F. (2002): Hyperglycemia increases endothelial superoxide that impairs smooth muscle cell Na+-K+- ATPase activity. Am. J. Phyiol. Cell Physiol., 282: 560-566.

Guyton, A.C. and Hall, J.E. (2006): Textbook of Medical Physiology. 11th ed. Philadelphia, PA: Elsevier Inc.

Haffner, S.M.; Lehto, S.; Ronnemaa, T.; Pyorala, K. and Laakso, M. (1998): Mortality from coronary heart disease in subjects with type 2 diabetes and in nondiabetic subjects with and without prior myocardial infarction. N. Engl. J. Med., 339: 229–234.

Hathout, E.H.; Sharkey, J.; Racine, M.; Thomas, W.; Nahab, F.; El-Shahawy, M. and Mace, J.W. (2000): Diabetic autoimmunity in infants and preschoolers with type 1 diabetes. Pediatric Diabetes, 1(3): 131-134.

Herzberg-Schäfer, S.; Heni, M. and Stefan, N. (2012): Impairment of GLP1-induced insulin secretion: role of genetic background, insulin resistance and hyperglycaemia. Diab., Obes. Metabol., 14:85–90.

HSG. (2008): Hyperglycemia and adverse pregnancy outcomes. New Engl. J. Med., 358: 1991-2002.

Huang, S. and Czech, M. P. (2007): The GLUT4 Glucose Transporter. Cell Metab., 5(4): 237–252

IDF. 2013. IDF Atlas. Available from: http://www.idf.org/diabetesatlas.

Imam, M. (2012): Clinical features, diagnostic criteria and pathogenesis. J. Adv. Exp. Med. Biol., 771: 340–355.

Inagaki, Y.; Yamagishi, S.; Okamoto, T.; Takeuchi, M. and Amano, S. (2003): Pigment epithelium-derived factor prevents advanced glycation end products-induced monocyte chemoattractant protein-1 production in microvascular endothelial cells by suppressing intracellular reactive oxygen species generation. Diabetologia., 46 (2):284-287.

Inoguchi, T.; Battan, R.; Handler, E.; Sportsman, J.R.; Heath, W.; Bursell, S. and King, G. (1992): Preferential elevation of protein kinase isoform II and diacylglycerollevels in the aorta and heart of diabetic rats: Differential reversibility to glycemic control by islet cell transplantation. Proc. Natl. Acad. Sci., 89:11059-11063.

Inoguchi, T.; Xia, P.; Kunisaki, M.; Higashi, S.; Feener, E.P. and King GL. (1994): Insulin's effect on protein kinase C and diacylglycerol induced by diabetes and glucose in vascular tissues. Am. J. Physiol., 267: 369-379.

Johnson, J.D. (2007): Pancreatic beta-cell apoptosis in maturity onset diabetes of the young. Canad. J. Diabetes, 31(1): 67-74.

Joseph, P. T. and Franck, M.-J. (2012): Importance of oestrogen receptors to preserve functional β-cell mass in diabetes. Nat. Rev. Endocrinol., 8: 342-351.

Kinoshita, J.H. (1990): A thirty year journey in the polyol pathway. Exp. Eye. Res., 50:567-573.

Kinoshita, J.H. and Nishimura, C. (1988): The involvement of aldose reductase in diabeti complications. Diabetes Metab. Rev., 4(4):323-337.

Ko, B.C-B.; Lam, K.S-L.; Wat, N.M-S. and Chung, S.S-M. (1995): An (A-C) dinucleotide repeat polymorphic marker at the 5'end of the aldose reductase gene is associated with earlyonset diabetic retinopathy in NIDDM patients. Diabetes, 44:727-732.

Koukkou, E.; Watts, G.F. and Lowy C. (1996): Serum lipid, lipoprotein and apolipoprotein changes in gestational diabetes mellitus: a cross-sectional and prospective study. J. Clin. Pathol., 49: 634-637.

Koya, D. and King, G.L.(1998): Protein kinase C activation and the development of diabetic complications. Diabetes, 47(6):859-866.

Kubo, E.; Maekawa, K.; Tanimoto, T.; Fujisawa, S. and Akagi, Y. (2001): Biochemical and morphological changes during development of sugar cataract in otsuka long-evans tokushima fatty (OLETF) rat. Exp. Eye Res., 73:375-381.

Kumar, P.J. and Clark, M. (2002): Textbook of Clinical Medicine. Pub: Saunders (London), 1099-1121.

Langer, O. and Conway, D.L. (2000): Level of glycemia and perinatal outcome in pregestational diabetes. J. Maternal-Fetal Med., **9** (1): 35-41.

Lee, A.Y.W. and Chung, S.S.M. (1999): Contribution of polyol pathway to oxidative stress in diabetic cataract. FASEB. J., 13:23-30.

Leng, Y.P.; Qiu , N.; Fang, W.J.; Zhang, M.; He, Z.M. and Xiong, Y. (2014): Involvement of increased endogenous asymmetric dimethylarginine in the hepatic endoplasmic reticulum stress of type 2 diabetic rats. PLoS. One, 9(2): 97125.

Leszek, S. (2011): Glucose Homeostasis – Mechanism and Defects, Diab.- Damages Treat., 978: 227-256

Lin, Y. and Sun, Z. (2010): Current views on type 2 diabetes. *Journal of* Endocrinol., 204:1-11.

Lindberg, G.; Lindblad, U. and Melander, A. (2004): Sulfonylureas for treating type 2 diabetes mellitus. Cochrane Database Systemic Reviews.

Lupachyk, S.; Watcho, P.; Stavniichuk, R.; Shevalye, H. and Obrosova, I.G. (2013): Endoplasmic reticulumstress plays a key role in the pathogenesis of diabetic peripheral neuropathy.Pathogen. diabet. Periph. Neuropa., 62(3) : 944–952.

Majithia, A. R. and Florez, C.J. (2009): Clinical translation of genetic predictors for type 2 diabetes. Current Opin. Endocrinol. Diab. Obes., 16(2): 100- 106.

Martin, A.O.; Simpson, J.L; Ober, C. and Freinkel, N. (1985): Frequency of diabetes mellitus in mothers of probands with gestational diabetes: possible maternal influence on the predisposition to gestational diabetes. Am. J. Obst. Gynecol., 151(4): 471-475.

Mathis, D.; Vence, L. and Benoist, C. (2001): Beta-Cell death during progression to diabetes. Nature, 414: 792–798.

Matsushita, K.; van der Velde, M.; Astor, B.C.; Woodward, M.; Levey, A.S.; de Jong, P.E.; Coresh, J. and Gansevoort, R.T. (2010): Association of estimated glomerular filtration rate and albuminuria with all-cause and cardiovascular mortality in general population cohorts: a collaborative meta-analysis. Chronic Kidney Disease Prognosis Consortium. Lancet., 12: 2073-2081.

Mauvais-Jarvis F.; Sobngwi, E.; Porcher, R.; Riveline, J.P.; Kevorkian, J.P.; Vaisse, C.; Charpentier, G. Guillausseau, P.J.; Vexiau, P. and Gautier, J.F. (2004): Ketosis-prone type 2 diabetes in patients of sub-Saharan African origin: clinical pathophysiology and natural history of beta-cell dysfunction and insulin resistance. Diabetes, Mar., 53(3):645-653.

Mauvais-Jarvis, F. and Kahn, C.R. (2000): Understanding the pathogenesis and treatment of insulin resistance and type 2 diabetes mellitus: what can we learn from transgenic and knockout mice? Diab. Metabol., 26, (6): 433-448.

McLarty, D.G.; Athaide, I.; Bottazzo, G.F.; Swai, A.M. and Alberti, K.G. (1990): Islet cell antibodies are not specifically associated with insulindependent diabetes in rural Tanzanian Africans. Diabetes Res. Clin. Pract., 9: 219-224.

McLellan, J.A.; Barrow, B.A.; Levy, J.C.; Hammersley, M.S.; Hattersley, A.T.; Gillmer, M.D. and Turner, R.C. (1995): Prevalence of diabetes mellitus and impaired glucose tolerance in parents of women with gestational diabetes. Diabetologia 38(6): 693-698.

Mellor, H. and Parker, P.J. (1998): The extended protein kinase C superfamily. Biochem. J., 332:281-292.

Metzger B.E. (1991): 1920 overview of GDM. Accomplishment of the last decade-challenges for the future. Diabetes, 40(2):1-2.

Mischenko, N.P.; Fedoreev, S.A. and Bagirova, V.L. (2003): Histochrome: A new original domestic drug. Pharm. Chem. J., 3: 48–52.

Mitchell, S.M. and Frayling, T.M. (2002): The role of transcription factors in maturity-onset diabetes of the young. Mol. Genet. Metab., 77: 35-43.

Neve, B.; Fernandez-Zapico, M.E.; Ashkenazi-Katalan, V.; Dina, C.; Hamid, Y.H.; Joly, E.; Vaillant, E.; Benmezroua,

Y.; Durand, E.; Bakaher, N.; Delannoy, V.; Vaxillaire, M.; Cook, T.; Dallinga-Thie, G.M.; Jansen, H.; Charles, M.A.; Clément, K.; Galan, P.; Hercberg, S.; Helbecque, N.; Charpentier, G.; Prentki, M.; Hansen, T.; Pedersen, O.; Urrutia, R.; Melloul, D. and Froguel, P. (2005): Role of transcription factor KLF11 and its diabetes-associated gene variants in pancreatic beta cell function. Proceed. Nati. Acad. Sci., 102(13): 4807-4812.

Nielsen, M.F. (2008): Contribution of defects in glucose production and uptake to carbohydrate intolerance in insulin-resistant subjects. Dan. Med. Bull., 55(2):89-102.

Noctor, G.; Arisi, A.M.; Jouanin, L.; Kunert, K.J.; Rennenberg, H. and Foyer, C.H. (1998): Glutathione: Biosynthesis, metabolism and relationship to stress tolerance explored in transformed plants. J. Exp. Bot., 49: 623–647.

Norris, J.M. and Rich, S.S. (2012): Genetics of glucose homeostasis: implications for insulin resistance and metabolic syndrome. Arterioscler. Thromb. Vasc. Biol., 329:2091-2096.

Nouwen, A.; Nefs, G.; Caramlau, I.; Connock, M.; Winkley, K.; Lloyd, C.E.; Peyrot, M. and Pouwer, F. (2011): Prevalence of depression in individuals with impaired glucose metabolism or undiagnosed diabetes: a systematic review and meta-analysis of the European Depression in Diabetes (EDID) Research Consortium. Diab. Care, 34: 752–762.

Obrosova, I.G. (2009): Diabetic painful and insensate neuropathy:

pathogenesis and potential treatments. Neurotherapeutics, 6: 638–647.

Pavy-Le Traon, A.; Fontaine, S.; Tap, G.; Guidolin, B.; Senard, J.M. and Hanaire, H. (2010): Cardiovascular autonomic neuropathy and other complications in type 1 diabetes. Clin. Auton. Res., 20: 153–160.

Perkins, J.M.; Dunn, J.P. and Jagasia S.M. (2007): Perspectives in gestational diabetes mellitus: a review of screening, diagnosis, and treatment. Clinical Diabetes, 25(2): 57- 62.

Phielix, E., and Mensink, M. (2008): Type 2 diabetes mellitus and skeletal muscle metabolic function. Physiol. and Behav., 94(2): 252-258.

Piciucchi, M.; Capurso, G.; Archibugi, L.; Delle Fave, M. M.; Capasso, M. and Delle Fave, G.; (2015): Exocrine pancreatic insufficiency in diabetic patients: prevalence, mechanisms, and treatment. Int. J. Endocrinol., 2015:595649.

Pischetsrieder, M. (2000): Chemistry of glucose and biochemical pathways of biological interest. Perit. Dial. Int., 20 (2): 26-30.

Porte, D.; Sherwin, R.S. and Baron, A. (2003): Ellenberg and Rifkin's Diabetes Mellitus. 6th ed. New York, NY: McGraw-Hill.

Poulsen, P.; Kyvik, K.O.; Vaag, A. and Beck-Nielsen, H. (1999): Heritability of type II (non- insulindependent)diabetes mellitus and abnormal glucose tolerance – a population-basedtwin study. Diabetologia., 42(2):139-145.

Proksch, P. and Muller, W.E.G. (2006): Frontiers in Marine Biotechnology. Horizon Bioscience: Norfolk, UK.

Ramana, K.V.; Chandra, D.; Srivastava, S.; Bhatnagar, A. and Srivastava, S.K. (2003): Nitric oxide regulates the polyol pathway of glucose metabolism in vascular smooth muscle cells. FASEB. J., 17:417-425.

Ridderstrale, M. and Groop, L. (2009): Genetic dissection of type 2 diabetes. Mol. Cellular Endocrinol., 297: 10-17.

Riguera, R. (1997): Isolating bioactive compounds from marine organisms. J. Mar. Biotechnol., 5:187-193.

Rowley, W.R. and Bezold, C. (2012): Creating public awareness: state 2025 diabetes forecasts. Popul. Health Manag., 15:194–200.

Saely, C.H.; Aczel, S.; Marte, T.; Langer, P. and Drexel, H. (2004): Cardiovascular complications in type 2 diabetes mellitus depend on the coronary angiographic state rather than on the diabetes state. Diabetologia., 47: 145-146.

Said, G. (2007): Diabetic neuropathy – a review. Nat. Clin. Pract. Neurol., 3: 331–340.

Schmidt, A.M.; Hori, O.; Bret,t J.; Yan, S.D.; Wautier, J.L. and Stern, D. (1994): Cellular receptors for advanced glycation end products: implications for induction of oxidant stress and cellular dysfunction in the pathogenesis of vascular lesions. Arterioscler. Thromb.,14: 1521–1528.

Schmidt, A.M.; Yan, S.D.; Stern, D.M. (1995): The dark side of glucose. Nat. Med., 1: 1002–1004.

Scollan-Kolippoulos, M.; Guadagno, S. and Walker E. (2006): Gestational diabetes management: guidelines to a healthy pregnancy. Nurse Practitioner, 31(6): 14-19.

Seki, M.; Tanaka, T.; Nawa, H.; Usui, T.; Fukuchi, T.; Ikeda, K.; Abe, H. and Takei, N. (2004): Involvement of brain-derived neurotrophic factor in early retinal neuropathy of streptozotocin-induced diabetes in rats: therapeutic potential of brain-derived neurotrophic factors for dopaminergic amacrine cells. Diabetes, 53: 2412-2419.

Selvarajah, D.; Wilkinson, I.D.; Emery, C.J.; Harris, N.D.; Shaw, P.J.; Witte, D.R.; Griffiths, P.D. and Tesfaye, S. (2006): Early involvement of the spinal cord in diabetic peripheral neuropathy. Diab. Care, 29: 2664–2669.

Sepe, S.J.; Connell, F.A.; Geiss, L.S. and Teutsch SM. (1985): Gestational diabetes: Incidence maternal characteristics and perinatal outcome. Diabetes, 34(2): 13-16.

Shiba, T.; Inoguchi, T.; Sportsman, J.R.; Heath, W.; Bursell, S. and King, G.L. (1993): Correlation of diacylglycerol and protein kinase C activity in rat retina to retinal circulation. Am. J. Physiol., 265: 783-793.

Shield, J.P. (2000): Neonatal diabetes: new insights into aetiology and implications. Hormone Res., 11: 537-511.

Shukla, N.; Angelini, G.D.; Jeremy, J.Y. (2003): Homocysteine as a risk factor for nephropathy and retinopathy in type 2 diabetes. Diabetologia., 46: 766-772.

Simmons, K. M. and Michels, A. W. (2015): Type 1 diabetes A predictable disease. World J. Diabetes, 6(3):380-390.

Singh, R.; Barden, A.; Mori, T. and Beilin, L. (2001): Advanced glycation end-products: a review. Diabetologia., 44: 129–146.

Sosale, A.; Saboo, B. and Sosale, B. (2015): Saroglitazar for the treatment of hypertrig-lyceridemia in patients with type 2 diabetes: current evidence. Diabetes Metab. Syndr. Obes., 8:189-196.

Staiger, H.; Machicao, F.; Fritsche, A. and Häing, H-U. (2009): Pathomechanisms of type 2 diabetes genes. Endocrine Reviews, 30(6): 557-585.

Stevens, M.J.; Dananberg, J.; Feldman, E.L.; Lttimer, S.A.; Kamijo, M.; Thomas, T.P.; Shindo, H.; Sima, A.A. and Greene, D.A. (1994): The linked roles of nitric oxide, aldose reductase and, (Na+, K+)-ATPase in the slowing of nerve conduction in the streptozotocin diabetic rat. J. Clin. Invest., 94(2):853-859.

Tangvarasittichai, S. (2015): Oxidative stress, insulin resistance, dyslipidemia and type 2 diabetes mellitus. World J. Diabetes, 6(3):456-480.

Tattersal, R.B. (1974): Mild familial diabetes with dominant inheritance. Quarterly J. Med., 43(170): 339-357.

Tattersal, R.B. and Fajans, S.S. (1975): A difference between the inheritance of classical juvenileonset and maturity-onset type diabetes of young people. Diabetes, 24(1): 44-53.

Tortora, G.J. and Grabowski, S.R. (2003): Principles of Anatomy and Physiology. 10th ed. New York, NY: Wiley.

UKPDS. (1998): Intensive blood-glucose control with sulphonylureas or insulin compared with conventional treatment and risk of complications in patients with type 2 diabetes (UKPDS 33). Lancet, 352: 837–853.

Unwin, N.; Gan, D. and Whiting, D. (2010): The IDF Diabetes Atlas: providing evidence, raising awareness and promoting action. Diabetes Res. Clin. Pract., 87: 2–3

Vinik, A.I.; Holland, M.T.; Le Beau, J.M.; Liuzzi, F.J.; Stansberry, K.B. and Colen, L.B (1992): Diabetic neuropathies. Diab. Care, 15: 1926–1975.

von Muhlendahl, K.E. and Herkenhoff, H. (1995): Long-term course of neonatal diabetes. New Eng. J. Med., 333(11): 704-708.

Wagaarachchi, P.T.; Fernand, L.; Premachadra, P. and Fernand, D.J.S. (2001): Screening based on risk factors in an Asian population. J. Obst. Gynecol., 21(1): 32-34.

Wallace, C.; Reiber, G.E.; LeMaster, J.; Smith, D.G.; Sullivan, K.; Hayes, S. and Vath, C. (2002): Incidence of falls, risk factors for falls, and fall-related factures in individuals with diabetes and a prior foot ulcer. Diab. Care, 25: 1983-1986.

Wardlaw, G.M. and Hampl, J.S. (2007): Perspectives in Nutrition. 7th ed. New York, NY: McGraw-Hill.

Watanabe, R.M.; Black, M.H.; Xiang, A.H.; Allayee, H.; Lawrance, J.M. and Buchanan, T.A. (2007): Genetics of gestational diabetes mellitus and type 2 diabetes. Diab. Care, 30(2): 134-.140.

Wessels, A.M.; Rombouts, S.A.; Simsek, S.; Kuijer, J.P.; Kostense, P.J.; Barkhof, F.; Scheltens, P.; Snoek, F.J. and Heine, R.J. (2006): Microvascular disease in type 1 diabetes alters brain activation: a functional magnetic resonance imaging study. Diabetes, 55: 334–340.

Wright, E.M.; Hirayama, B.A. and Loo, D.F. (2007): Active sugar transport in health and disease. J. Int. Med., 261:31-43.

Yabe-Nishimura, C. (1998): Aldose reductase in glucose toxicity: a potential target for the prevention of diabetic complications. Pharmacol. Rev., 50(1):21-33.

Zimmet, P.; Cowie, C.; Ekoe, J.M. and Shaw, J.E. (2004): Classification of diabetes mellitus and other categories of glucose intolerance. In: International Textbook of Diabetes Mellitus chapter 1, 3rd Ed., 3-14.

ABOUT THE AUTHOR

Dr. Ayman Saber Mohamed was born in Giza, Egypt, in 1984. He received the B. Sc.degree in chemistry and zoology from faculty of science, Cairo University, Egypt, in 2011. He joined the Department of zoology, Faculty of science, Cairo University as a Demonstrator in 2013. In 2014, he got the M. Sc.degree and became teacher assistant of molecular and integrated physiology.